HOW TO BEAT INSOMNIA

Francisco Javier Alguacil Rodríguez

PRESENTATION

This book contains demonstrated advances and techniques on the best way to deal with all the regions of Insomnia from the causes to the means on the best way to fix it. All the data in this book will assist you with conquering the cycle of Insomnia.

All the evenings of remaining wakeful and all the times of continually feeling depleted will disappear.

In the wake of perusing this book, you will know about where Insomnia comes from, however you will likewise realize how to fix it.

Much appreciated again and I trust you appreciate this book and advantage hugely from it!

PART 1: THE SCIENCE BEHIND INSOMNIA

Have you ever experienced a sleeping disorder? At the end of the day, do you face the trouble of nodding off and staying unconscious around evening time?

So what causes it? Intermittently, a sleeping disorder is brought about by numerous reasons, for example, not getting enough rest, hunger, mental injury, etc.

Regardless of what the explanation is, a large number of people experience the ill effects of the demon called a sleeping disorder.

It burglarizes you from getting enough rest, saps your energy and annihilates your efficiency the following day.

Also the un favorable impact towards your own physical and emotional well-being.

What is Insomnia?

A sleeping disorder by definition is the trouble of nodding off and staying unconscious.

It alludes to the kinds of anxiety an individual endures at various purposes of their rest cycle.

A straightforward sign to analyze sleep deprivation is the point at which an individual isn't happy with the measure of rest that the person in question has been getting.

Those with sleep deprivation will feel the absence of energy, weariness at various snapshots of the day, confronting trouble in focusing on errands, encountering awful mind-set aggravations, and having a low-execution level in the work environment.

It's feasible for sleep deprived people to have any of these side effects subsequent to remaining wakeful for the duration of the evening.

A human body expects rest to revive both brain and body. An absence of rest in both of them will bring about weakness and different dysfunctional behaviors.

In spite of the fact that they are horrendously depleted deeply, they actually neglect to nod off or stay unconscious because of various causes.

The two Types of Insomnia

1. Intense Insomnia: There are two primary sorts of a sleeping disorder. The main sort is the sort of sleep deprivation when you just endure a few eager evenings.

Intermittently, you're ready to nod off and stay unconscious without any problem.

For some, sleep deprived people probably won't imagine that they are experiencing it yet the truth of the matter is, they could be having Acute Insomnia. So what is Acute Insomnia? This sort of sleep deprivation comes from the center degrees of stress that restless people are encountering at that point.

They will confront a brief period where they can't nod off due to the existence conditions they're looking at that point.

This kind of a sleeping disorder doesn't keep going for a delayed time. All things considered, it just occurs because of specific variables or occasions during a predetermined timeframe.

For example, intense a sleeping disorder may happen after restless people confronted the rage of their chief, gotten a terrible evaluation on a test, got dismissed by their squash, or only on the grounds that they're having a "Awful Day".

These circumstances can make an individual have an evening or two where the person basically can't get any rest. Numerous individuals may have encountered this sort of a sleeping disorder and it will in general purpose all alone.

2. Constant Insomnia: The second sort of a sleeping disorder is known as Chronic Insomnia. It's a delayed sort of a sleeping disorder which happens in any event three evenings for each week and goes on for at any rate three months.

Typically, this happens when you are confronting a critical change in your current circumstance, truly or intellectually.

It very well may be moving to another home, losing a friend or family member, being in another working environment, confronting difficulties in school, or experiencing difficulty adjusting to a harsher climate.

Maybe, the motivation behind why ongoing restless people are experiencing difficulty with rest is that they have an unfortunate rest propensity without an appropriate rest schedule.

It's regular in this day and age; current culture has botched rest cycle with brief long stretches of rest. To exacerbate the situation, the majority of them rest at odd hours.

They don't rehearse the propensity for hitting the sack early and rising promptly the following day.

Therefore, the brain doesn't have a clue when to close down and would be acquainted with keeping awake until late.

That is the motivation behind why sleep deprivation has become a typical issue in the present society.

What individuals neglect to comprehend is that the body won't have the option to work with a limited quantity of rest one evening and hope to repay their rest hole by taking snoozes later on during the day.

While this may appear to be conceivable and help full before all else, this rest design isn't feasible as long as possible.

In the end, the psyche and body will implode, and you will encounter total depletion until you get enough rest.

The best fix is to have a fixed timetable to rest and practice sound rest schedule.

Else, you need to visit the specialist for drug. Ordinarily it will be connected to another clinical or mental issue; implying that the motivation behind why you may be having persistent a sleeping disorder will be because of stress.

What is by all accounts a run of the mill circumstance will appear to be upsetting on the off chance that you have ongoing a sleeping disorder.

An eager brain and body will feel irritated by any improvement from the quick climate.

The Causes of Insomnia

Notwithstanding the sorts of a sleeping disorder, the causes are the equivalent. The distinction lies in the force of feelings an individual encounters for a set measure of time. Other than that, fundamental ailments can likewise cause sleep deprivation. Luckily, sleep deprivation is treatable by and large.

These ailments can be either extreme or gentle, prompting sleep deprivation to happen at an alternate point in an individual's life.

These indications incorporate nasal sensitivities, sinus hypersensitivities, lower back torment, generally speaking constant torment, gastrointestinal issues, joint inflammation, asthma, and other neurological issues.

The weight on the patient's body will make the brain stay conscious for a more extended timeframe.

For example, the individuals who contract a bug will understand that they are remaining wakeful for most of the evening or they may end up awakening regularly.

Both of these elements can bring about an individual having an extreme absence of rest and rest. They may attempt to unwind while having a cold, however sleep deprivation will win.

Actual agony can likewise cause a sleeping disorder as the body can't get into an agreeable situation to rest.

Have you ever experienced restless evenings since you can't get into an agreeable position? The present circumstance is run of the mill when you experience any torment in your body.

The most ideal approach to nod off and stay unconscious quick is to get your body in an agreeable situation in bed.

It will likewise help in mending and guarantee a more profitable rest. Else, you'll wind up in a consistent fight to nod off and even pick pointless medicine in the event that you can't get into your best dozing stance.

In light of these various causes, we would now be able to proceed onward to the fix.

In any case, it's similarly as essential to concentrate all the elements that cause sleep deprivation. Yet, did you realize that there are likewise hazard components of a sleeping disorder? On the off chance that you discover a portion of these dangers concern you, at that point you basically have a higher possibility of having a sleeping disorder sooner or later in your life.

Something else, focus on your wellbeing and rest propensities to ensure that you're sleep deprivation free for the remainder of your life.

The Risk Factors of Insomnia

The danger variables of a sleeping disorder incorporate being a female, being pregnant or in the time of menopause, grown-ups over the age of forty, experiencing more pressure, experiencing melancholy, make some night memories work, travel significant distances where there is a period change, or have a family background of a sleeping disorder.

These elements lead an individual nearer to sleep deprivation. In any case, do you understand that a large portion of these danger factors are the consequences of your decisions? By and large, individuals feel that they have practically zero decision throughout everyday life, which isn't correct.

They can decide to take a more drawn out get-away when they are traveling through various time regions, yet they didn't.

They can go for a normal everyday employment, except they chose to experience the tough situations of having a work around evening time and adjust to a completely unique way of life.

It is difficult to manage the danger elements of sleep deprivation, at the end of the day everything relies upon your decisions.

At times, you may experience difficult stretches throughout everyday life. It tends to be relationship issues, family issues, or occupation issues.

Not just that, you may be experiencing monetary or individual issues where you are experiencing difficulty adjusting your expert and individual life.

All these will pummel you and keep you up around evening time until the majority of the pressure or melancholy is no more. At times, it may take longer. In different cases, individuals can discover arrangements and overcome the difficult stretches rather rapidly.

In any case, having the correct attitude is the fix to feelings initiated sleep deprivation. Since sleep deprivation has a wide range of causes and danger factors, there are various things that you can do to keep yourself from having more restless and eager evenings.

More often than not, it's not difficult to discover what the causes are, yet the genuine test is the means by which to defeat it and have a decent night rest.

Life can be troublesome, and some of the time it can thrash an individual to where he's not even sure on the off chance that he can get back up.

The absolute initial phase in beating sleep deprivation is to be intrepid. Try not to be frightened of any results or results that may or probably won't occur.

Dread achieves more pressure in your life that doesn't serve you. Indeed, it can just increase your a sleeping disorder. Counteraction is in every case in a way that is better than fix.

Continuously make sure to remain quiet and follow the wellbeing tips to keep yourself from having a sleeping disorder.

PART 2: THE BRAIN OF AN INSOMNIAC

Scientists all around the globe are assembling their psyches to sort out how the mind of a sleep deprived person works. They keep on looking towards the highlights of the multitude of brainwaves and how the contemplations collaborate during the day and night.

How the Mind Works

During all day long, the psyche can adjust to any new circumstance. Regardless of whether you're attempting to get food, get a beverage, escape the vehicle, strolling through an entryway, or simply get some rest, the psyche will continually attempt to discover better approaches to endure and thrive.

It will proceed through the pattern of getting enough assets during the day and have enough energy to mend and rest during the evening.

Typically, individuals with a sound degree of brainwaves with agreeable psychological dependability during the day can close down pieces of the cerebrum's perspective during the evening.

As dusks further, the mind will start to back off and start rest. Your sharpness and concentrate normally decline when it's evening. This is the motivation behind why an individual thinks that it's harder to finish any errands around evening time.

Studies show that the cycle of the psyche will normally change for the duration of the day, and at times it will cause a significant type of uneasiness.

It is the point at which the brainwaves become inconsistent and decline to back off because of a gigantic measure of pressure during the day. Along these lines, the psyche won't have the option to unwind totally around evening time.

All things being equal, it will experience a period where the brainwaves will move strangely quick, causing more musings and burning-through more energy at night.

All that an individual has experienced during the day will be recalled around evening time.

The body will at that point go through double the measure of energy and assets to handle the musings, and this causes exhaustion and absence of energy the next day.

The Mind and the Brainwaves

Concerning the psyche and how the brainwaves react to the periods of sleep deprivation, there are three distinct investigations to show how the cerebrum responds during the evening.

It has demonstrated that the cerebrum's learning and memory preparing capacities influence an individual's rest.

The more you pick up during the day, the more considerations and recollections will be handled by the cerebrum during the evening. Dreams come from one's contemplations and genuine encounters.

The more you experience throughout everyday life, the more you dream around evening time.

The capacity to have a bigger assortment of dreams permits the psyche to quiet down and frame ambiguous pictures to fortify your memory.

At the point when you fall into profound sleep, you will in general be in the fantasy state.

Now and again, you may even have bad dreams.

However, everything reduces to your subliminal contemplations and the sort of involvement you had.

Day Vs Night

So what's going on in the mind of sleep deprived people? First and foremost, their mind is more dynamic during the evening and experiences issues in getting to the without a care in the world state.

In one of the investigations on the brainwaves during sleep deprivation, researchers have demonstrated that the neurons of the restless people's mind are more dynamic around evening time.

Light sleepers will in general have a ton of considerations experiencing their head which brings about sleep deprivation.

They're encountering a consistent condition of data handling all through the whole day without the capacity to end it.

At last, they'll have a sleeping disorder and face the outcomes of not having enough rest. Specialists guarantee that sleep deprivation ought not be seen straightforwardly as an evening time disorder.

In certainty, it's to a greater degree a 24-hour cerebrum condition that makes the mind stay dynamic for the duration of the day.

Rest assumes a significant part in preparing and putting away recollections. The absence of rest will meddle with your memory over the long haul.

You'll experience difficulty concentrating, recalling realities, and even minor subtleties. This hypothesis was tried out with a gathering of understudies on a short test.

One gathering had an entire night rest though another gathering didn't have any rest the prior night.

The outcomes? Understudies who had more rest had the option to concentrate more, and they had the option to review their answers of the test a couple of hours after the fact.

The gathering of understudies who needed more rest battled with the test, scored less than ideal, and barely reviews the appropriate responses they composed an hour after the test!

The Myths

The objective of this investigation is to demonstrate the significance of rest to an individual's concentration and memory.

In actuality, sleep deprived people can't have a similar degree of focus as the individuals who had enough rest.

Shockingly, a few people accept that they can have a similar capacity to focus during the day.

Because the cerebrum is as dynamic around evening time all things considered during the day, it doesn't imply that the mind can work at the pinnacle level.

Other than the absence of fixation, research shows that Insomniac has more cerebrum versatility.

Nonetheless, the examination on what pliancy is and how it adds to the conditions of sleep deprivation is at this point unclear.

However, what they can be sure of is that the versatility of the cerebrum develops all through an individual's life, and adds to different types of illness later on.

Mind pliancy is the capacity of the cerebrum to change fundamentally and practically because of physical or natural factor.

As a rule, cerebrum pliancy empowers us to retain new data, learn new things, and keep on developing all through adulthood.

However, in case of a sleeping disorder, it harms your synapses and prompts cerebrum versatility.

This prompts helpless memory maintenance and absence of core interest.

In a momentary premise, however in the long haul also.

It is additionally testing to clutch all the degrees of focus and memory when an individual becomes more seasoned.

The Brain of the Restless Mind

Another examination was never really out what stress and tension mean for rest. The objective was to decide if an individual with an unpleasant way of life has a sleeping disorder, and how the mind reacts around evening time.

What's more, here's the outcome: The psychological capacity of the cerebrum doesn't change notwithstanding they have sleep deprivation, or not.

Nonetheless, restless people think that it's additionally testing to center and deal with data for the duration of the day. Most exploration shows that the psyche of restless people meanders during the evening.

They will experience issues thinking the following day; they'll face difficulties in dealing with their work, considers and even their own lives.

As such, the brain will think that it's hard to work ideally the following day and restless people can't perform at their best.

Another piece of the examination analyzed the memory work and the productivity to finish any errands given to sleep deprived people and to the individuals who had enough rest.

Studies show that restless people can't remember a large portion of their recollections during the day.

Therefore, they face trouble in finishing their day by day errands. Their psyches would meander in any event, when they're performing straightforward assignments.

For instance, with regards to getting ready breakfast, those with a sound measure of rest will go to the kitchen, settle on snappy decisions, and start their day.

Then again, those who're experiencing sleep deprivation will enter the kitchen, wind up opening more cupboards, glancing through similar nourishments, and incapable to sort out what they ought to have for breakfast!

What's more, here's the clarification: A restless person's brainwaves are slower, and this will make the person in question move at a more slow speed and fail to remember basic things rapidly.

Besides, as they go on during that time and as more errands come their direction, the prefrontal cortex will start to have less assets, and the brainwaves will get inconsistent.

The cerebrum will attempt to remain dynamic, yet it won't have enough energy to deal with everything. Hence, the cerebrum will debilitate itself ultimately in case you're experiencing a sleeping disorder.

The Gray Matter

The third and last logical examination is to decide the job of the cerebrum's dark issue. The main thing to think about the gray matter is that it exists in the frontal flap and controls the cycles of memory and chief capacity.

At the point when restless people don't get enough rest around evening time, they

Will have a considerable abatement in dark issue. Regardless of whether they are experiencing sleep deprivation or experiencing difficulty dozing by and large, they will begin to create manifestations of despondency or injury gradually.

Generally, the basic reason for a sleeping disorder is pressure. The most ideal approach to determine this issue is to counsel a specialist to discover what sort of medication would be best for you.

Basically, the psyche needs to acquire enough rest and rest to have a satisfactory fixation.

Sleep deprivation will just place your body into overdrive mode and accordingly not be getting enough rest.

The following significant thing to recollect is to get enough nourishment and rest each night.

Regardless of the fact that it is so hard to track down an equilibrium, it is essential to have an undeniable degree of fixation consistently to take advantage of your day.

PART THREE: SLEEP STARVED - THE DEVIL

In the last section, the psyche was investigated to see what a sleeping disorder straightforwardly means for the cerebrum. Having this issue for any measure of time will cause an enormous negative effect on the brain.

Other than cognitive decline, a sleeping disorder additionally brings about sluggishness, indiscretion, and absence of sharpness the following day.

The psyche and body both need rest to work well the following day. In the event that there is no rest, at that point the dark issue, memory, and expand obligations of the brain will disintegrate, and light sleepers will struggle traversing the day.

Their brain will meander, and they will battle to remain centered for the duration of the day.

The 5 Things You Do Every Morning

Here's a little exercise: Firstly, attempt to consider all the things you did the second you awaken today.

Think about the initial five things that you did. You may kill the morning timer, check the telephone, stand up, switch on the lights, and stroll to the restroom.

Regardless of what your standard routine is, you will in general execute all your ordinary exercises impeccably. In all honesty, you subliminally play out every one of these exercises without really thinking about, simply because it turned into a day by day schedule.

Be that as it may, when you have sleep deprivation, you are not close to as engaged as you ordinarily are.

The psyche will keep on deduction as fast as it typically would, yet it doesn't have all the assets and energy to work appropriately.

All together words, you may think that it's hard to play out your initial five exercises toward the beginning of the day, and battle to finish each errand.

A simple method to realize this is the point at which you understand that it took longer than it should when playing out these errands.

The five activities that should require just 2 minutes finishing may wind up requiring over 10 minutes when you needed more rest. You may even neglect to do an assignment or two.

You may neglect to kill the caution, and you may neglect to check your telephone for any updates.

Various things can occur, yet generally this is just a glimpse of something larger when you are battling with a sleeping disorder.

Harming Your Professional Life

After the primary evening confronting sleep deprivation, you may see a huge drop in your energy level.

You may see that it's hard to design the day, or you may think that its additionally testing to recollect all the data during the day.

As a rule, your day by day schedule may start with awakening, preparing for work, or even go out to shop thereafter.

All positions require 100% concentration to guarantee superior and effectiveness.

Else, you may recognize the cold hard reality from your chief.

Regardless of how depleted you may feel, there are just a specific measure of days that you will be given compassion.

There are just so many debilitated leaves you can require in a year. So don't allow sleep deprivation to pulverize your own and expert life.

Assume responsibility and dispose of it for the last time. In your work, you are required to finish the undertakings before a specific cutoff time.

Regardless of whether you are accountable for pressing boxes, doing research, or composing, you must be at the highest point of your game consistently.

You need to perform at your best constantly and acquire your merited check toward the month's end.

Any rest forfeited during the night can bring about lackluster showing the following day.

Is it true that you are Experiencing Sleep starved?

Everybody has their exceptional rest cadence, and specialists suggest 6-8 hours rest day by day.

The specific number relies upon the person. A few of us need more rest, some less.

Be that as it may, toward the day's end, losing several hours of rest is in every case in a way that is better than losing an entire evening of rest.

For example, rather than getting eight hours of rest, you just get six hours of rest. Those two hours of rest may appear to be essential, yet they won't harm your life as a sleeping disorder.

Losing two hours of rest may back you off, yet risks are, you will in any case ready to get it through and complete all the errands before the days over.

Then again, losing a whole evening of rest can close your mind down. They will experience the day battling with basic errands.

For example, when your manager puts a plan around your work area, you can peruse the substance without an issue.

Yet, acknowledging what everything on the rundown implies is the interesting part for those with sleep deprivation.

What is by all accounts a stroll in the recreation center may seem like mission unimaginable for restless people.

Periodically, you lose center and reason for the afternoon in the event that you need rest. You'd be continually searching for the quickest method to traverse the day instead of pondering the most ideal approach to get past the day.

Initially, it may appear to be reasonable on the grounds that you're as yet ready to complete things on time sometimes.

Yet, truly, it'll hurt your standing in your working environment over the long haul in light of the fact that the low quality of your work.

Additionally, sleep deprived people are known to have terrible temper and helpless working relationship with their partners.

Individuals will see your failure at last. Your manager will see that you are working at a slower rate, that you are not centering so a lot, and that you don't have the correct disposition to finish the work.

It can place you in some unacceptable courtesy of your chief, and you may likewise hazard being terminated.

Albeit this may appear improbable to you at the present time, you should remember that the chance is high.

Sleep deprivation is an upsetting component to life that not ex-

clusively can raise somebody ruckus in the working environment
yet in addition in their own life.

Harming Your Personal Life

At the point when you consider your own life, consider all that are critical to you, things that you hold truly to your heart.

You may consider your better half, spouse, youngsters, pets, or some other viewpoints.

A few people may even consider their nursery or their rebuilding project that they have been chipping away at.

There is no correct response to this. It's your own life, and the way to accomplishment in your own life is to look after adjust.

A great many people play out their day by day schedule without placing a lot of thought into it.

Models are straightforward assignments, for example, planning breakfast for your children, getting into the vehicle, or heading off to some place to eat. Typically, these aren't troublesome undertakings, yet restless people may feel in any case.

The second an individual's very own life begins to get off equilibrium, it brings about upsetting minutes, and they start to address if there is any approach to return to the consistent state.

It doesn't make a difference if the pressure is coming from not having some staple goods as expected or getting up late, an insignificant measure of pressure can amass into something that is crazy.

A sleeping disorder causes a lot of pressure and fatigue.

There won't be particular contemplations in their brain; their psyche will just meander with arbitrary considerations without setting.

The equivalent can likewise be applied to their work life. On the off chance that you are experiencing sleep deprivation and you need to set up your children for school, you may miss the lunch box, neglect to press their garments, and the rundown goes on.

Continuously make sure to put yourself first as "Self esteem isn't Selfish". At the point when you continually set yourself last, you'll wind up in a descending twisting of life, incapable to satisfy your definitive reason throughout everyday life.

Right now is an ideal opportunity to totally expose an enormous misguided judgment in our general public, the view of putting yourself first as haughty, evil, and narrow minded.

What they neglected to comprehend is that in case you're occupied with satisfying the requests of others while not accomplishing your life purposes, you'd feel unfulfilled and damned.

You'd lose your drive, inspiration, eagerness, and profitability on the off chance that you venture down this way. So quit satisfying others and focus on yourself first.

Exclusively thusly you'll have a relentless energy to achieve more, and have more to bring to the table consequently.

At home, you may have to keep up your home by trimming the grass or strolling around the house to check for bugs.

Regardless of what you do, you need to recall the means to execute each activity precisely.

The second you are experiencing a sleeping disorder, you won't have the option to recall things well indeed, and you will make some harder memories completing it.

Another crucial piece of your own life is your relationship with others.

Regardless of whether it's your accomplice, spouse, wife, beau, or sweetheart, being seeing someone a work all alone.

In the event that you neglect to give full consideration to your accomplice since you needed more rest, at that point you can anticipate that your relationship should turn sour.

The present circumstance will prompt contentions, disappointment, dissatisfaction, depression, and bitterness in a relationship. These feelings can go so astray to where significant encounter may have to occur.

Managing Insomnia

It's difficult to manage a sleeping disorder when you have no energy left inside you. You'll feel tired constantly and care less about things that are occurring around you.

Your psyche will meander, and intermittently those contemplations don't bode well. Life itself is as of now hard enough.

Presently, envision including the way that you are not getting any rest and need to manage each impediment life present you.

How might you feel? Overpowered? Focused? You may wind up sitting around at your work environment.

You may neglect to set up your family dinners and upset your kids. You may begin overlooking all the seemingly insignificant details that you as a rule accomplish for your sentimental relationship. Numerous regions in your day to day existence can go south because of a sleeping disorder.

In light of all these, right now is an ideal opportunity to shield you from losing rest and get ideal rest each night.

PART 4: THE CURE: NATURAL AND ARTIFICIAL REMEDY

Rest is staggeringly significant for wellbeing. We need rest for our body to recuperate and revive from our day's exercises.

Tragically, numerous individuals either experience issues nodding off or essentially don't get enough rest, which is the place where Insomnia cures come in.

There are two essential classes with regards to Insomnia Remedies.

Counterfeit Remedy

The first is the Artificial Remedy. This kind of cure or medication can be found in the drug store and center. They are typically endorsed to focus on the infection at the source.

Fake cure ordinarily costs a bomb, yet it normally conveys quick outcomes. Most medication today is poisonous, loaded up with unsafe synthetics that are undependable to be burned-through for a drawn out timeframe.

Normal Remedy

The other sort of cure is called Natural Remedy. Individuals have rehearsed characteristic medication for quite a long time. This kind of cure uses the body's regular mending measure for beating sleep deprivation.

It is frequently more affordable; however what makes them stand apart is the way that they're not as harmful as Artificial Remedy.

Despite which sort of cure you pick, the objective is to help you nod off and stay unconscious.

These cures are intended to help you to get more rest around evening time. The vast majority of these cures will cause languor, so it's ideal to take them just before bed except if it states in any case.

It is likewise imperative to ensure that you converse with a specialist prior to getting any medicine recorded beneath.

- Eszopiclone: Also known as Lunette, is a gathering of medications fit for taking care of you effectively and rapidly.

Insights show that Lunette is can take care of the vast majority for a normal of 7-8 hours.

It's a solid gathering of medications, so ensure you avoid it except if you're ready to have an entire night rest to forestall drowsiness. FDA restricts the medication measurement to be not more than 1mg.

Anything else than that may bring upon the danger of tiredness the following day.

- Ramelteon: This gathering of medications works in an unexpected way, it doesn't make unfavorable impacts the clients, for example, languor, tiredness, etc.

Basic medications used to prompt rest focuses on the CNS (Central Nervous System), discouraging its capacities and put the client in a drowsy state.

Ramelteon, then again, targets explicitly the rest wake cycle. This medication is endorsed to the individuals who experience issues nodding off. Because of the absence of results, Ramelteon can be endorsed for long-term use. The medication has additionally indicated no set of experiences of misuse or reliance.

- Zaleplon: Also known as Sonata. Most medications have a long enactment time in a human body.

Sonata isn't one of them. Among all the most recent resting pills, Sonata figured out how to remain dynamic in the framework for the briefest measure of time.

As such, this medication leaves practically zero results the following morning. For example, if an individual experiences issues nodding off, a fly of Sonata pill will help him nod off without feeling off the following day.

- Doxepin: Also known as Splendor. This gathering of medications is endorsed explicitly to the individuals who experience issues staying unconscious.

You can say that this is a counterfeit solution for the "light sleepers" who effectively awaken around evening time because of a negligible measure of boosts.

It acts by smothering the histamine receptors, along these lines helping your rest upkeep after you've nodded off.

As this medication expects you to stay unconscious for a set measure of time, don't burn-through Splendor except if you're ready to snooze for full 7-8 hours around evening time.

The measurement relies upon your reaction to treatment, well-being, and age.

- Benzodiazepines: Benzodiazepines are helpful for both present moment and long haul a sleeping disorder.

It lastingly affects the body as it stays in the framework for quite a while. Along these lines, for those who've had sleep deprivation for quite a while, this medication can help them in their excursion to full recuperation.

It's regularly used to treat delayed bad dreams and sleepwalking. As the impact of this medication is steady, you may feel drained and lazy the following day. Another symptom of this prescription is that this medication can bring about medication reliance, implying that you may need to depend on this medication to nod off and stay unconscious in future.

Benzodiazepines can be found in dozing pills Triazolam (Halcion), Alprazolam (Xanax), Temazepam (Restoril), and others.

It is imperative to get a clinical assessment before you take any resting pills. Visit a specialist for a careful assessment.

Continuously counsel your primary care physician about the unfriendly impacts of any medicine prior to choosing which pills to take.

Each medication can cause diverse results. The results can be a cerebral pain, extreme unfavorably susceptible response, drawn out tiredness to simply name a couple.

Then again, some would like to go for regular cures all things considered.

You don't need to rely upon synthetic compounds with unsafe antagonistic impacts particularly after awakening. All things considered, why not utilize regular solutions for fix your rest cycle and shut down a sleeping disorder.

Go Camping

At the point when the draw of the TV or playing on the telephone keep you up late around evening time, it's an ideal opportunity to get the tent and go outdoors.

Avoid electronic gadgets and appreciate an advanced deter sometimes. Put yourself in an interruption free zone and be aware of your environmental factors and yourself.

Use this opportunity to contemplate, do some yoga, compose, recall your musings, or just relax. As indicated by a few investigations, campers who avoid contraptions and work on slowing down customs, for example, ruminating or tuning in to music nodded off around 2 hours sooner than expected.

Another significant highlight recollect is that advanced gadgets add to insomnia. It is discovered that counterfeit light sources can contrarily influence circadian rhythms.

Give resting a shot the ground, not in your vehicle or lodge. That way, you'll get grounded and be unified with nature.

Notwithstanding what you do during outdoors, a definitive objective is to unwind, eliminate yourself from interruptions and requests from others, to avoid fake light, and be unified with nature.

Shower under the characteristic daylight and nod off when the sun goes down. Right away by any means, you'll reset your rest rhythms.

Music Therapy

Music has been utilized since old occasions to battle sleep deprivation. It is a recuperating device that can assist with facilitating tension which can add to helpless rest quality.

The significant preferred position of this method is that it's not difficult to utilize and has no result. There are a wide range of kinds of music treatments, and they contrast in the sorts of neurological incitement they inspire.

For example, old style music can be an integral asset for solace and unwinding while exciting music may cause uneasiness.

Attempt to go for delicate loosening up music that has hints of nature like the sea, feathered creatures, cascade, and so forth.

A few investigations demonstrated that individuals who tune in to quieting music prior to hitting the sack had improved rest quality during the night than individuals who don't. Henceforth, in case you're experiencing difficulty nodding off, this could be an answer.

Shut Down For Better Sleep

Rest is anything but an on-and-off switch. Your body needs an ideal opportunity to loosen up and prepared itself for shuteye.

Sleep deprived people regularly think that it's hard to close off their cerebrum around evening time.

You can attempt to shut down for better rest. This method helps in calming things down so your body will comprehend that it's an ideal opportunity to get some rest.

To make way for rest, it is important to loosen up and faint our brain.

For example, on the off chance that you take a warm before sleep time, it'll make a drop in internal heat level, setting off the body to begin preparing for rest.

By washing up, your internal heat level will hinder metabolic capacities like breathing, assimilation, and pulse.

Your body will comprehend that it's an ideal opportunity to back off and unwind.

On the off chance that you have the propensity for tuning in to music prior to going to bed each night, your body will be molded that tuning in to music around evening time signals sleep time.

It's about propensities and molding. Cut out at any rate thirty minutes of wind-down time before bed to do breathing or un-winding activity to clear your brain.

The objective of this shut down hour is to flag your mind that it's an ideal opportunity to slow down, unwind and rest.

Rest in a Cool Room

Those who've issue nodding off ordinarily have a higher center internal heat level promptly earlier nodding off when contrasted with their better partners.

Accordingly, this gathering of restless people needs to sit tight for in any event 2 to 4 hours before their internal heat level brings down and starts rest.

Exploration shows that the ideal room temperature for rest is between 16 to 20 degrees Celsius.

At the point when you're attempting to rest, your cerebrum appreciates the chilly climate. Moreover, resting in a cool room likewise helps in enemy of maturing.

It helps in delivering of against maturing chemicals known as melatonin, an intense cell reinforcement that handles irritation, fortifies the insusceptible framework, and forestalls psychological weakening and disease.

There's a maxim that the individuals who hit the sack early and rise early live more. It bodes well thinking about that resting in a cool room diminishes neuron-degeneration and oxidative pressure.

I can continue endlessly with respect to the counter maturing advantages of having a decent night rest in a cool climate.

In any case, the way to upgrading the creation of hostile to maturing chemicals in your body is to have a satisfactory rest.

What's more, the initial step to do that is to establish an ideal dozing climate by bringing down the room temperature. Inadequate rest carries a great deal of unsafe impacts to your physical and psychological wellness.

At last, it can put your life in danger. So make a point to fix your resting propensities, and you can start doing as such by establishing an ideal dozing climate.

Start to Sweat

Exercise early. It's a well known fact that activity improves rest and by and large wellbeing. Yet, an investigation distributed in the diary Sleep shows that the sum of activity done and when they exercise have an effect.

Analysts found that ladies who practice at a moderate force for in any event 30 minutes every morning, 7 days per week, experience less difficulty dozing than ladies who practice less or later in the day.

Morning exercise appears to decidedly influence our body rhythms that thus improve our rest quality.

One reason for this exchange among exercise and rest might be internal heat level. Your internal heat level ascents during activity and requires as long as 6 hours to drop down to typical.

This is on the grounds that cooler internal heat levels connect to all the more likely rest. So it's essential to give your body time to chill off before bed.

Rest is a critical piece of our wellbeing and mending. Pay attention to it, and search out the assistance of a useful medication professional on the off chance that you can't get your rest leveled out.

All these require order and responsibility. When you reset your organic clock and fall once again into the typical rest mood, you'll at long last appreciate the advantages of serene, therapeutic rest.

PART 5: LIFESTYLE MODIFICATION
FOR INSOMNIAC

In the past part, we discussed the two basic classes of solutions for defeat a sleeping disorder. Notwithstanding, these extraneous components couldn't manage the base of a sleeping disorder. Indeed, you can feel better subsequent to evaluating those cures, yet a sleeping disorder must be mended totally if the cause of the issue is eliminated.

Something else, there is a high possibility for sleep deprivation to backslide. So what is the foundation of sleep deprivation? For some, the essential driver of a sleeping disorder is having a helpless way of life and rest propensities.

Basic way of life changes can improve things significantly to the nature of your rest.

Albeit not all a sleeping disorder is brought about by stress, but rather it is verifiable that individuals who experience continuous pressure are more helpless to sleep deprivation.

On account of stress related a sleeping disorder, treating or killing the pressure will reduce a sleeping disorder. As referenced in the prior part of this book, stress influences the nature of one's rest which can agitate their rest beat.

Subsequently, one will think that it's hard to nod off around evening time and stay wakeful during the day.

It is essential to deal with all pieces of your life in the most ideal way to guarantee that you are at a good arrangement.

You need to ensure that you are getting adequate rest consistently. Rest assumes a significant part in your actual wellbeing. Inadequate rest for a brief timeframe may make you more grouchy and bad tempered.

Long haul impacts can be not kidding: cardiovascular issues, sadness, stroke, coronary failure, to give some examples.

As indicated by rest specialists, a few examinations demonstrated that when individuals get adequate rest, they won't just feel much improved, however will likewise expand their chances of living longer, better, and more refined lives.

To defeat a sleeping disorder, you should avoid any nicotine, caffeine, and liquor. These will make the brain become eager extra time normally.

Having a consistent measure of caffeine will compel the brain to be more dynamic than it is. A great many people need the energy to begin their day, so they picked energizer.

Caffeine is perhaps the most famous decisions of energizer today to guarantee sharpness and alertness toward the beginning of the day and for the remainder of the day. In any case, they're uninformed to the way that caffeine is one of the main sources of sleep deprivation.

It botches the characteristic equilibrium of alertness and rest. Consequently, restless people should avoid these beverages to have a quality rest.

Avoid that short breather, go after a glass of plain water rather than the espresso, which might be the motivation behind why you are experiencing difficulty falling and staying unconscious around evening time.

Other than that, setting up a rest plan for you is outstanding amongst other self improvement procedures for a sleeping disorder.

It is a significant advance in defeating a sleeping disorder for good.

It is so essential to hit the hay simultaneously around evening time and wake up a similar time each day on the grounds that the body needs consistency.

The body loves a daily schedule. It blossoms with propensity. With a standard sleep time and wake-up time, your body is bound to remain on target.

In the event that you can, try not to substitute timetables, late night parties, night shifts or different things that may upset your rest plan.

At the point when you struggle nodding off, attempt to drink a glass of warm milk. It is a customary solution for a sleeping disorder, and there's proof that it can assist you with improving quality rest.

In addition to the fact that milk helps keep hunger from upsetting your rest, however it additionally contains an amino corrosive called tryptophan, which is changed over in the mind into an "unwinding" synthetic known as serotonin.

Calcium is supportive of metabolic, lessening pressure and diminishing degrees of parathyroid chemical, which has been known to assume a part in sleep deprivation.

Not simply that, you can generally change your own day by day timetable to incorporate time for yoga or contemplation.

There is a bounty of proof that yoga and reflection can improve rest designs, regularly significantly. Possessing some unwinding energy for you is significant.

These methods should be possible at home for both solace and security. It assists with expanding the all out adaptability of your body, loosen up your mind and distress your body.

Attempt to go through in any event 30 minutes per day to either reflect or yoga. Normally contemplation and yoga are best done in the early morning, in a peaceful spot and with openness to daylight.

For reflection, you should simply plunk down and clear your brain. Attempt to tune in to loosening up music to help quiet you down.

The second you begin to become accustomed to reflecting for the duration of the day, the brain will have the option to loosen up quicker around evening time and hence you will make some simpler memories nodding off.

Concerning yoga, you can either go for yoga classes with a lot of companions or practice at home for more security.

It will profit your rest from multiple points of view. The act of certain yoga stances will expand the blood flow to the rest community in the cerebrum, which has the impact of normalizing the rest cycle.

Keep in mind, rest isn't a direction for living or an extravagance; it is regular and vital.

So root out the hidden causes, change your eating routine, drink a glass of warm milk, set up a dozing plan, do some yoga and ponder.

Follow the suggestions referenced above, and in the long run, you'll get your quality rest.

PART 6: SWITCHING OFF

Doing combating Insomnia

Battling sleep deprivation is a daunting task. At the point when you are attempting to fix a sleeping disorder, you are really attempting to prevent your psyche from being excessively dynamic around evening time.

There is no motivation to fear keeping awake for endless evenings in succession and contemplating whether it is all going to end. Stressing will just bring over restless evenings.

So quit engaging sleep deprivation in your mind! That you should simply "Switch-Off" your monkey cerebrum.

Around evening time, you need your psyche to back off to where you can rapidly nod off.

Having an appropriate measure of rest encourages you to remain completely alert the following day, and guarantees a decent night rest.

One reason why individuals battle to nod off is on the grounds that their monkey cerebrum will not close down.

As a rule, they begin contemplating pointless things that fill no need except for just impede them from nodding off. Turning off requirements practice.

For some bustling grown-ups, the lone time they consider their lives is during sleep time!

It's acceptable to reflect sometimes, yet not during sleep time.

In many cases, this is the greatest offender that prevents you from nodding off.

So for the individuals who need to think about their lives, consider getting up prior to have time toward the beginning of the day to do as such or even timetable some time at night to do some reflection.

Animating Night = Bad Sleep

Another motivation behind why individuals neglect to turn off is that they have numerous exercises around evening time that are over animating, making them stay conscious as opposed to feeling tired.

Some even love to have caffeine around evening time!

No big surprise individuals are battling to nod off! So avoid espresso, from your cell phones, workstations, TVs when it's sleep time.

Stay away from exercises that constrain you to think and require actual effort around evening time.

Furthermore, above all, evade 'Blue-screen' from the electronic gadgets.

Never Miss another Night of Sleep

Another key to nod off is to plan your rest. A great many people don't do that. All things considered, they decide to nod off just when they're drained.

However, what they ought to do rather is to set up their everyday practice and timetable their sleep time.

Upon reiterations, your psyche will be molded to turn off when the clock hits the typical hour to nod off.

Having a standard rest routine is apparently the best strategy to guarantee a superior quality rest.

Indeed, our bodies blossom with predictable rest timetable and consistency. In spite of the fact that there's nobody size-fits all arrangement, having a steady rest routine will help in beating constant sleep deprivation unequivocally.

The most effective method to "Switch-Off" at Night

The main thing you ought to do after you have had supper and tidied up for the night is turn off any of your electronic gadgets.

Having your telephone or PC turned on when you are preparing for bed will invigorate your cerebrum and it will in the end prevent your rest.

Let it be known, your electronic gadgets are addictive, and you won't realize when to stop.

The light will meddle your rest example and cause you to remain wide alert. It's prescribed to try not to utilize your contraptions no matter what at any rate 1 hour before sleep time.

Perusing before rest is fine, yet not through your electronic gadgets. Perusing an actual book as a diversion before bed really encourages you in preparing to rest.

It's better not to peruse in your room. You're urged to peruse in another room since you don't need your psyche to be dynamic in the room that you need to nod off in.

Once more, to condition your brain to turn off the second you venture into your room. On the off chance that you can totally loosen up when perusing a book, at that point it's fine to do it while setting down in bed.

Something else, it's ideal to peruse in another room. The following thing you can do is tune in to music and record any sort of updates that you will require for the following day.

The music will assist you with quieting your brain and eliminate your pressure away. Attempt to tune in to music that is smoother and slower in mood. Tuning in to anything that is boisterous or energizing will invigorate the psyche, and it will be more enthusiastically for you to nod off.

For occurrence, you'll wind up in a much-loosened up state when you tune in to old style music than awesome music. Another tip is to prepare before rest.

Recording updates for the following day assists with getting out your brain. Remaining alert in bed while continually advising yourself that you need to recollect something will keep your psyche dynamic.

Consider your scratch pad a "dump it and fail to remember it" vault. Just get a piece of paper and scrawl a couple of notes down. It will help you quiet down and nod off quicker. Something else that you can do is having an unwinding drink, for example, tea just before bed.

Nonetheless, ensure that you avoid caffeine, liquor, and beverages with a high measure of sugar. A pleasant cup of tea can quiet your psyche down and causes your body to unwind. This is additionally a magnificent method to make time for you.

A chance to calm down and unwind. You can do this while either perusing or tuning in to music.

On the off chance that you don't discover joy in drinking tea, at that point consider having a light nibble before bed. Try not to devour whatever is too high in calorie and hard to process.

Notwithstanding, a light tidbit is acceptable on the grounds that occasionally, the motivation behind why you're experiencing difficulty having the opportunity to rest is basically because of appetite.

Another approach to guarantee serene rest is to cut down your room temperature. The most ideal approach to do this is to set your room indoor regulator to be somewhat cooler. Our body is molded such that when it enters a cooler climate, it will get a sign that it's an ideal opportunity to rest. Additionally, why not clean up just before bed.

Ideally a virus shower to promptly chill off. Else, you can attempt to get a bed fan, cooler bedding, or take a short stroll before bed.

Everything recorded above can be a piece of your sleep time schedule.

Feel free to give them a shot and figure what turns out best for you and your timetable. Quickly by any means, you won't experience any difficulty nodding off and staying unconscious once more.

Final Conclusion

I trust this book can serve and guide you in halting or forestalling sleep deprivation.

You're allowed to attempt any tips and methodologies recorded in this book to guarantee a relaxing rest.

All things considered, relaxing rest is the establishment for your psychological and actual prosperity.

Regardless of whether it's counterfeit or common cure, way of life changes, or setting up a daily practice, all these add to forestalling sleep deprivation.

So what to do straightaway? It's an ideal opportunity to make a move today! Discover which of these techniques turn out best for you and actualize them into your every day schedule.

Record them and envision how your normal day appears as though when you add these procedures to your daily schedule.

Simply by giving them a shot, you can discover the most ideal path for you to defeat sleep deprivation.